AF802641

MULTISKILLING:

Team Building

FOR THE HEALTH CARE PROVIDER

ACKNOWLEDGMENTS

Appreciation is extended to the following individuals and health care organizations for their assistance and support in developing this module:

Clarian Health Partners, Inc., Indianapolis, Indiana
Tony Beverly, Maintenance Technician, Facilities
Sammy Booker, Zone Service Worker, Facilities
Neddra Griffen, Zone Service Worker, Facilities
Donald Mathis, Zone Service Worker, Facilities
Don Weir, Senior Training Consultant, Educational Services
St. Vincent Hospital, Indianapolis, Indiana
Joan Barr, RN, Director, 3 South and Coronary Intensive Care Unit
Rita Emerick, RN, MSN, Senior Development Consultant to Educational Services
Diana Graham, MSN, CNS, NP, Development Consultant to Educational Services
Bonnie Hiner, RN, Practice Facilitator, Coronary Intensive Care Unit
Barbara Bloom Kreml, BBK & Associates, Chicago, Illinois

Appreciation is expressed to the following practitioners and educators for their critical reviews of the manuscript.

Sharon Dykes, RN, BSN, MSA, Three Rivers Community College, Poplar Bluff, Missouri
Beverly M. Kovanda, PhD, Columbus State Community College, Columbus, Ohio
Perka Kresic, MS, MT (ASCP), Trocaire College, Buffalo, New York
Sally Stafford Lewis, MS, H, HTL (ASCP), Tarrant County Junior College, Hurst, Texas
Earl P. Murphy, Dean, Allied Health Sciences, Trident Technical College, Charleston, South Carolina
Delores J. Pederson, RN, BSN, Albuquerque Technical Vocational Institute, Albuquerque, New Mexico
Claire Teske, RN, BA, Shasta-Trinity ROP, Redding, California

MULTISKILLING:

Team Building

FOR THE HEALTH CARE PROVIDER

Sherry Makely, PhD, RT(R)
Director, ADD-A-COMP® Program, and
Manager, Employee Education and Development
Clarian Health Partners, Inc.
Indianapolis, Indiana

Beverly M. Kovanda
PhD, MS, MT (ASCP), CLP (NCA)
Series Editor

Delmar Publishers

an International Thomson Publishing company ITP®

Albany • Bonn • Boston • Cincinnati • Detroit • London • Madrid
Melbourne • Mexico City • New York • Pacific Grove • Paris • San Francisco
Singapore • Tokyo • Toronto • Washington

Cover Design: Scott Keidong's Image Enterprises

Delmar Staff

Publisher: Susan Simfenderfer
Acquisition Editor: Dawn Gerrain
Developmental Editor: Marjorie A Bruce
Project Editor: Brooke Graves/Graves Editorial Service
Team Assistant: Sandra Bruce

Art and Design Coordinator: Vincent S. Berger
Production Coordinator: John Mickelbank
Marketing Manager: Katherine Slezak
Marketing Coordinator: Glenna Stanfield
Editorial Assistant: Donna L. Leto

Printed in the United States of America

For more information contact:
Delmar Publishers
3 Columbia Circle, Box 15015
Albany, New York 12212-5015

International Thomson Publishing Europe
168–173 Berkshire House
High Holborn
London, WC1V7AA
England

Nelson ITP, Australia
102 Dodds Street
South Melbourne,
Victoria, 3205 Australia

Nelson Canada
1120 Birchmount Road
Scarborough, Ontario
M1K5G4, Canada

International Thomson Publishing France
Tour Maine-Montparnasse
33 Abenue du Maine
75755 Paris Cedex 15, France

International Thomson Editores
Seneca 53
Colonia Polanco
11560 Mexico D. F. Mexico

International Thomson Publishing GmbH
Königswinterer Strasse 418
53227 Bonn
Germany

International Thomson Publishing Asia
60 Albert Street
#15–01 Albert Complex
Singapore 189969

International Thomson Publishing—Japan
Hirakawa-cho Kyowa Building, 3F
2-2-1 Hirakawa-cho, Chiyoda-ku,
Tokyo 102, Japan

ITP Spain/Paraninfo
Calle Magallanes, 25
28015-Madric, Expana

2 3 4 5 6 7 8 9 10 XXX 03 02 01 00 99

ISBN: 0-8273-8524-2

MESSAGE FROM THE SERIES EDITOR

The Multiskilling for Health Care Providers series consists of the *Patient Care: Basic Skills for the Health Care Provider* core text and many separate modular texts. The Multiskilling series offers a comprehensive vision of the diversity and many implications of multiskilling, whether in an acute care setting, home care, hospice, ambulatory setting, long-term care facility, or physician's office. The core text and module subjects have been identified through research as key topics in multiskilling and patient care training across the nation.

The framework for this series is found in the historic evolution of multiskilling, the National Health Care Skill Standards, and 13 years of personal experience in developing academic materials and successfully training thousands of multiskilled health care providers in a multitude of nursing and allied health skill areas. The concept referred to as *multiskilling*, *cross-training*, and (more recently) *patient care skills* began to gain national awareness in the mid-1980s, as pressures for cost containment in health care intensified. Institutions began to focus on more efficient use of personnel for economic survival. The implications of managed care are far-reaching.

In 1994, the National Health Care Skill Standards were developed through a national collaborative effort of health care organizations, professional organizations, schools, and colleges of higher education. By implementing these standards, we can more effectively serve the needs of a diverse client population and maintain quality care, while increasing the efficiency of staff utilization. Health care costs can be contained; the new technology, which is changing how and where health care is delivered, can be prudently applied. We believe that the skill standards are important and so their intent has been incorporated into the entire series.

The core text, *Patient Care: Basic Skills for the Health Care Provider*, meets the OBRA requirements for basic patient care skills. These skills are required of every health care provider who undertakes client care, regardless of the institutional setting or professional affiliation.

We believe that the core-text-plus-modules concept is the only rational approach to meeting the vastly different academic and training needs in multiskilling, as we re-engineer careers in all health care settings. The modules are flexible, well written, and academically sound. The modular approach is cost-effective. A health care worker's skills can be developed based upon individual goals, institutional needs for retraining, or specific career development. Colleges, hospitals, other health care agencies, technical and career schools, and "tech prep" programs need only purchase the modules that address their unique, customized academic and training needs. Because multiskilling is market-driven, other modules continue to be developed as health care needs are identified and evolve.

The modules are written by credentialed experts in each content area and multiskilling education. They have identified essential and appropriate nursing and allied health skills that can be accurately and safety performed by nonprofessionals to enhance the quality of patient care.

The depth of theory and skills in each module goes beyond other texts, which are usually written from the perspective of one profession rather than by specialists in each identifiable allied health and nursing area. We believe that this principle provides a stronger basis for instruction and facilitates a higher level of quality patient care.

The material in each module is organized in a clear, concise, straightforward manner to make learning easier, because health care institutions are demanding shorter—but intensified—training periods. The pedagogical features enhance retention and simplify learning.

We believe that the Multiskilling series combines the knowledge, experience, successes, and expertise of all of the authors. It provides the tools and flexibility to custom-design a curriculum that truly meets worker/student professional goals, augments valuable skills, and strengthens employability, not only now but as we prepare for the 21st century.

Beverly M. Kovanda, PhD, MS, M.T. (ASCP), CLP (NCA)
Coordinator/Professor, Multicompetency Health Technology
Columbus State Community College, Columbus, OH

DELMAR'S MULTISKILLING SERIES

Patient Care: Basic Skills for the Health Care Provider
Multiskilling: Advanced Patient Care Skills for the Health Care Provider
Multiskilling: Phlebotomy Collection Procedures for the Health Care Provider
Multiskilling: Electrocardiography for the Health Care Provider
Multiskilling: Respiratory Care for the Health Care Provider
Multiskilling: Point of Care Testing—Capillary Puncture for the Health Care Provider

Modules Coming Soon:

Multiskilling: Waived Laboratory Testing for the Health Care Provider
Multiskilling: Team Building for the Health Care Provider
Multiskilling: Health Unit Coordination for the Health Care Provider
Multiskilling: Rehabilitation Services for the Health Care Provider
Multiskilling: Dietary Assisting for the Health Care Provider

TABLE OF CONTENTS

PREFACE

It's an exciting new world in health care and team skills have never been more important. Whether you work directly with patients or provide clerical or support functions in a hospital or outpatient setting, the ability to function as an effective team member is a critical key to success. Maybe you are just starting your career in health care and need to know more about teams and how they function. Or perhaps you have been working in health care for some time and have recently been retrained or cross-trained for a new, team-based job. In any case, this module will help you gain a better understanding of team dynamics and the skills you need to be an effective team member.

Multiskilling: Team Building for the Health Care Provider covers the "who," "what," "when," "where," and "why" of health care teams, and most important, the "how": how to be an effective team member yourself. This module describes different types of teams, explains why some teams work well whereas others do not, and details personal and team characteristics required for success.

Each chapter includes Review Questions (with Recommended Responses provided in the Appendix), and Suggested Learning Activities for individuals and groups. A list of Supplemental Resources to further enhance learning is provided at the end of the module.

CHAPTER 1

Traditional Teams in Health Care

OBJECTIVES

After reading this chapter, you will be able to:

- *List five common activities of traditional health care teams.*
- *Define the terms teamwork, intradisciplinary, interdisciplinary, intradepartmental, interdepartmental, homogenous, heterogeneous, work teams, and project teams.*
- *List, describe, and give two examples of six different types of traditional health care teams.*

■ ***teamwork:*** *two or more people combining individual efforts toward a common goal*

OVERVIEW

This chapter describes six different types of teams traditionally found in health care, and the kinds of activities they commonly perform.

Teamwork has always been important in health care as physicians, nurses, technologists, therapists, and clerical and support personnel work together in pairs or in groups of three or more people to care for patients, and provide a wide variety of health-related services. In general, teams typically:

- work together to perform job duties
- coordinate work assignments
- share information and resources
- organize special projects
- set standards and monitor outcomes
- recommend quality improvements
- develop policies and procedures
- test and evaluate new technology
- identify training needs

Today's rapidly changing health care system calls for even more emphasis on teams and teamwork than in the past. Before exploring new types of teams, team-based jobs, and what you can expect as a team member yourself, let us first take a look at traditional types of teams in health care.

There are at least three different ways of categorizing traditional teams in health care. Each categorical grouping is based on the types of workers involved, and the purpose or mission of the team itself.

INTRADISCIPLINARY AND INTERDISCIPLINARY TEAMS

■ ***intradisciplinary:*** *within a discipline*

Intradisciplinary teams are composed of workers from the *same* discipline. Team members all have similar training, job titles, scopes of responsibility, and levels of expertise. Because of such similarity, intradisciplinary teams are also referred to as **homogeneous** teams. Sometimes, intradisciplinary team members all work in the same department; other times they do not. For example, registered nurses from several patient care units might participate on a team to develop new charting procedures, home health aides might meet each morning to coordinate patient visits, insurance claims processors in a physician group practice might work as a team to expedite financial reimbursement, or teams of secretaries might test new computer software.

■ ***homogeneous:*** *composed of similar characteristics*

Interdisciplinary teams are composed of workers from *different* disciplines. Team members may have different training, job titles, scopes of responsibilities, and levels of expertise. Because of such differences, interdisciplinary teams are also referred to as **heterogeneous** teams. Interdisciplinary team members might or might not all work in the same department. A team of registered nurses and dietitians might meet regularly to monitor the progress of diabetic patients. Radiographers, laboratory personnel, and admitting clerks might form a team to streamline inpatient pre-admission testing. Or a team of housekeeping, maintenance, and risk management workers might meet monthly to address cleanliness and safety issues.

■ ***interdisciplinary:*** *between or among two or more different disciplines*

■ ***heterogeneous:*** *composed of different characteristics*

INTRADEPARTMENTAL AND INTERDEPARTMENTAL TEAMS

Intradepartmental teams are composed of workers from the *same* department. An intradepartmental team might include a group of phlebotomists, medical laboratory technicians, and medical technologists charged with reducing the cost of laboratory supplies. A team of pharmacists might work together to select new drugs for use in their hospital. In an outpatient clinic, a team of medical assistants might meet bimonthly to arrange continuing education sessions for the rest of the staff.

■ ***intradepartmental:*** *within a department*

Interdepartmental teams are composed of workers from two or more *different* departments. A team might be composed of emergency room personnel, cardiac catheterization technologists, and surgical nurses who work together to devise methods of assessing heart attack victims and getting them into surgery more quickly. Or therapists, therapy assistants, and rehabilitation technicians from the occupational therapy and radiation therapy departments might meet regularly to coordinate the care and rehabilitation of cancer patients.

■ ***interdepartmental:*** *between or among two or more different departments*

WORK TEAMS AND PROJECT TEAMS

Work teams typically meet on a regular and on-going basis as an integral part of their jobs. At the beginning of each shift, teams of registered nurses, licensed practical nurses, and nurse assistants might meet to exchange patient information and coordinate work assignments. A team of operating room schedulers and transportation department personnel might meet early each morning to ensure that patients arrive on time for surgery. And a team of admitting department personnel and financial analysts might meet regularly to compare inpatient census rates with monthly projections.

■ ***work teams:*** *groups of individuals working together on a daily, on-going basis as an integral part of their regular jobs*

Unlike on-going work teams, **project teams** are typically short-term teams. Project teams are composed of groups of workers assembled to accomplish specific goals within an established period of time. A team of workers from nursing, central supply, and materials management might meet regularly during a one-month period to compare the use of disposable versus nondisposable patient supplies. A team of environmental services workers might be given two months to test a new disinfectant and report the results. Or medical assistants, infection control personnel, and public health workers might serve on a team for six months to identify options for improving air quality in a community neighborhood health clinic.

■ ***project teams:*** *groups of individuals working together for a defined period of time to accomplish specific goals*

These examples represent a few ways to categorize the different types of teams traditionally found in health care. As you have probably realized, category definitions and examples of each overlap. Regardless of how we describe them, health care simply would not be the same without teams. In Chapter 2, we will see why teams and teamwork are even more important today than in the past.

REVIEW QUESTIONS

1. Which of the following are common activities of traditional health care teams?
   _____work together to perform job duties
   _____coordinate work assignments
   _____share information and resources
   _____set standards and monitor outcomes
   _____identify training needs
   _____all of the above
   _____none of the above
2. Define the following terms, and give one example of each as it applies to a type of health care team: intradisciplinary, interdisciplinary, intradepartmental, interdepartmental, homogenous, and heterogeneous.
3. Describe the difference between a work team and a project team , and give one example of each.

SUGGESTED LEARNING ACTIVITIES

1. Think back to the last time you received health care services. Describe the location and setting (physician's office, clinic, emergency room, or hospital). List the different types of personnel who worked there. What role did each person play individually? How did the group function as a team? Did the group's work appear well organized? Why or why not? Describe some individual characteristics and behaviors that contributed to, or detracted from, the spirit of teamwork. If you worked in that setting, what improvements would you suggest to enhance teamwork?
2. Invite a health care supervisor or manager to be a guest speaker at your class, or arrange a time to interview such a person at his or her place of work. Find out what role teams have traditionally played in the organization, and how much responsibility teams have. What kinds of workers participate on teams? Are the workers patient caregivers, or do clerical and support staff also work on teams? Are teams homogeneous or heterogeneous? Categorize each team based on the different examples given in this chapter. What types of activities do the teams perform? How do teammates interact with one another? What role does the team leader play? How does one team interface with other teams? What skills do team members need to be successful?
3. Select a crossword puzzle and give each group member a copy. Complete the puzzle individually, and record the total number of words each person identified. Then collaborate as a group on the same puzzle. Record the total number of words the group identified together. Who was more successful? One individual working alone or the entire group working together?
4. Set up a survival scenario such as the Subarctic Survival Situation or the Mountain Adventure (see "Supplemental Resources" at the end of this module: refer to Human Synergistics International for the **Subarctic Survival Situation** and to **Games Teams Play** for the Mountain Adventure). After completing the exercise, compare individual success with team success and discuss the results.
5. Arrange a scavenger hunt as a team competition. Develop a list of 30 items for the scavenger hunt, and determine a prize or reward for every member of the winning team. Tell participants there is no limit to the number of people who can be on a team, and there is no limit to the total number of teams participating. Let the group divide up into teams any way they choose. Provide each team with a copy of the list, and give them 15 minutes to find as many of the 30 items as possible. When the time expires, add up how many items each team found, and determine which team's total is the highest. Distribute the prizes or rewards to each member of the winning team. Discuss the rationale behind how and why the group divided up into teams the way it did. Did the process work well or could it have been better? Ask

participants how it feels to be "winners" or "losers." Do the winners feel good about their prizes or rewards, even though the others in the group lost? How do the losers feel about the winners? Discuss competition versus teamwork, and review the rules of the exercise. Was there a way that everyone could have won so there would have been no losers? If they had worked together as one team, could they have found more items during the fifteen-minute timeframe than any single team did?

CHAPTER 2

New Roles for Health Care Workers

OBJECTIVES

After reading this chapter, you will be able to:

- *Define the terms specialist, hospital restructuring, work redesign, cross-training, multiskilled, and extenders.*
- *Describe the organizational structure of hospitals until the mid 1980s.*
- *Explain why many hospitals have decided to restructure within the last ten years.*
- *List two benefits of employing multiskilled workers.*
- *Give three examples of multiskilled clinical, clerical, and support workers.*
- *Give two examples of patient care extenders.*
- *Explain how restructuring, work redesign, and multiskilling impact the roles of health care workers.*

OVERVIEW

This chapter describes how teams and teamwork are changing because of the impact of hospital restructuring, work redesign, and multiskilling, all of which lead to drive the reorganization of who does what, and how and where they do it. Topics include the traditional organizational structure of hospitals, why and how many hospitals have restructured in recent years, and the roles of specialists, multiskilled workers, and patient care extenders.

ORGANIZATIONAL RESTRUCTURING OF HOSPITALS

Until the mid 1980s, the organizational structure of hospitals had remained largely unchanged. Hospitals were divided into different departments, each providing a distinct set of patient tests, treatments, or support services. Departments were separate from one another, and from nursing units where patients were housed. The majority of hospital staff worked in one department and functioned as **specialists**. Their education and work experience focused on a single discipline such as nursing, respiratory care, physical therapy, cardiovascular diagnostics, or radiography. Support staff specialized in food service, patient transportation, housekeeping, central supply, or maintenance work. Other personnel specialized in patient admitting, financial billing, insurance processing, medical records, and secretarial work.

■ ***specialists:*** *workers who provide one function, or a set of similar functions, in one discipline*

By 1984, however, mounting financial pressures caused hospitals to search for new ways to offer services at lower cost. Based on recent research, some investigators determined that the traditional way of structuring hospitals was just too expensive and inefficient to meet budgetary challenges. The "walls" that separated departments and nursing units caused workers and patients to travel long distances to complete tests and treatments, and unnecessary time was spent organizing logistics and waiting for elevators and transportation aides. Therefore, **hospital restructuring** became commonplace as organizations

■ ***hospital restructuring:*** *reorganizing the configuration of departments and work units in a hospital to change the way patient care and health services are provided* started to experiment with new ways of delivering patient care. As a result, a new approach, called patient-focused or patient-centered care, emerged.

Patient-focused care radically restructured operations. Services such as phlebotomy and EKG, traditionally based in two different departments, were "decentralized" and moved to patient care units. Soon afterwards, other services were decentralized as well, and patients could receive most of the tests, treatments, and support services they needed without ever having to leave their units.

WORK REDESIGN AND MULTISKILLING

■ ***work redesign:*** *reorganizing tasks and worker roles to change job responsibilities*

■ ***cross-training:*** *acquiring new, additional skills in the same discipline or in a different discipline as a worker's original skills*

■ ***multiskilled workers:*** *personnel who have been cross-trained to provide more than one function, often in more than one discipline*

To support this new approach to providing care, hospitals incorporated **work redesign** into their plans. Each job was examined to see how well it fit into the new structure, and some new roles emerged. Employers reconsidered exactly how much training and expertise a worker actually needed to perform a specific function. As a result, some responsibilities were re-assigned.

Increasing numbers of employers also began **cross-training** workers to produce more flexible, cost-effective personnel. Clinics, physician practices, and small and rural hospitals had cross-trained workers for years as a strategy to avert financial difficulties. By the mid 1980s, hospitals and health facilities of all types, sizes, and locations began to adopt the same concept.

Cross-training creates **multiskilled workers**: people who can provide more than one function, often in more than one discipline. As a result of restructuring, work redesign, and cross-training, many employees no longer work in one department doing one specialized job. Nurses may be cross-trained to draw blood, perform EKG testing, and give routine respiratory treatments. Radiographers, who once worked only in radiology departments may now be assigned to a satellite x-ray facility on a patient care unit, or may be cross-trained to do basic laboratory testing and help nurses with patient assessments. Unit secretaries may be cross-trained to do patient admitting, medical coding, and financial billing. And housekeepers may perform basic maintenance duties, order and stock inventory supplies, and transport patients.

In recent years, multiskilling has become a major trend. Medical assistants working in clinics or physician practices may be cross-trained to perform ultrasound procedures and help with outpatient surgery. Clerical workers in outpatient facilities are acquiring patient care skills, and caregivers are learning clerical functions. Increasing numbers of tests and treatments are now available in long-term care facilities and in patients' homes. People working in those settings are becoming cross-trained to perform additional functions as well.

If you have been working in the health care field for some time, you have probably encountered the trend toward multiskilling. Perhaps you have been notified that cross-training has become an expectation of your job. And if you are just starting your career, you may find that cross-training is a condition of employment. In any case, the demand for multiskilled workers is growing, and workers who are versatile and possess multiple skills benefit from enhanced employment opportunities.

Although multiskilling is on the rise, specialists are still needed in health care. In fact, specialists will always play a vital role in caring for patients and providing a variety of health-related services. However, today's changing environment calls for fewer specialists and more multiskilled workers.

EXTENDERS

■ ***extenders:*** *personnel with limited expertise and scopes of responsibilities who assist in the work of other personnel with greater expertise and broader, higher scopes of responsibilities*

Another aspect of work redesign and multiskilling involves the increasing use of **extenders**, people with limited training and skills who work under the supervision of personnel who are more highly educated and experienced, and often licensed. Nurse extenders, sometimes called patient care assistants or patient care technicians, are usually multiskilled. Although job responsibilities vary from place to place, they may include functions such as phlebotomy, EKGs, patient transport, vital signs, and other basic patient care procedures. Nurse practitioners and physician assistants are examples of physician extenders. And rehabilitation technicians are extenders for physical and occupational therapists.

In Chapter 3, we will discuss the impact of organizational restructuring, work redesign, and multiskilling on teams and teamwork.

REVIEW QUESTIONS

1. Define the following terms and give one example of each: specialist, hospital restructuring, work redesign, cross-training, and multiskilled worker.
2. Describe the organizational structure of hospitals up to the mid 1980s.
3. Explain why many hospitals have decided to restructure within the last ten years.
4. List two benefits of employing multiskilled workers.
5. Give one example of a multiskilled clinical worker, clerical worker, and support staff worker.
6. Define the term extender and give two examples.
7. Explain how restructuring, work redesign, and multiskilling impact the roles of health care workers.

SUGGESTED LEARNING ACTIVITIES

1. Identify a hospital in your community that has recently undergone organizational restructuring. Invite a manager to meet with your class, or arrange a time to visit the hospital. Find out when, why, and how the hospital reorganized. What were the goals of reorganization, and how does the new structure compare with the old? Was work redesign part of the plan? If so, why were jobs redesigned? How did worker roles change? Did only patient caregivers have their jobs redesigned, or were clerical and support staff also affected? Were people cross-trained? If so, what are some examples of multiskilled workers? Are any types of extenders used? If so, how do they fit into the staffing plan? Has the role of teams and teamwork changed as a result of restructuring? How do teams in the new environment compare with those of the past? Are job titles, performance appraisals, and pay increases connected with teams and teamwork? Using categories of teams previously discussed, what types of teams work in this restructured hospital? How much responsibility do teams have? What skills are necessary to function effectively? Where is the hospital headed in terms of future restructuring, work redesign, multiskilling, and use of extenders and teams?
2. Interview at least three different health care workers from the same hospital, including a patient caregiver, a clerical worker, and a support staff member. Find out how their jobs have changed, or are expected to change, as a result of restructuring. Do they have new job titles? Were they cross-trained, retrained, or reassigned to a different department? Are they working on one or more teams? If so, what kinds of teams, and what are the teams' responsibilities? How do the workers feel about their new roles, and what are the pro's and con's? What are the future prospects for their hospital and their jobs? What advice would they offer others preparing for jobs in health care?
3. Make a list of the different types of behaviors that occur when people try to work together in groups. Decide which behaviors are appropriate and inappropriate, and why. Which behaviors help groups accomplish their goals, and which ones impede success? Which behaviors support a spirit of teamwork and mutual respect and which do not? Using this list, identify "norms" for your group: standards of conduct that guide and control proper and acceptable behavior to help ensure the group's success. Consider that:
   - each person is expected to participate in group discussions
   - each person should have the opportunity to voice his or her opinion
   - no individual or group of individuals should dominate the discussion
   - everyone's opinions should be respected, even when others don't agree
   - all opinions should be taken into consideration before a decision is made
   - individuals should be willing to compromise to help the group reach an agreement.

   Think carefully about these group norms, and take them into consideration each time a team activity is undertaken.

4. Identify which characteristics and outcomes make an effective team, and develop a rating system to evaluate team effectiveness. Consider factors such as:
   - all group members participate openly and honestly
   - each individual has the opportunity to voice his or her opinion
   - all members feel respected by others in the group
   - the group is able to reach agreement within a reasonable period of time
   - the workload is shared equally among group members
   - leadership roles are well defined and shared among group members
   - the group completes tasks appropriately and on time

   Each time you participate in a team activity, rate the group's effectiveness based on these characteristics. What works well, and what needs improvement?

5. Videotape a group discussion or team meeting. Replay the tape and discuss what you have observed. Were group norms followed? Why or why not, and what impact did this have? Rate the effectiveness of the group. What worked well, and what needed improvement? If the group meets on an on-going basis, videotape future meetings and continue to observe, evaluate, and make improvements. Videotape several different group discussions or team meetings and compare them. Did different groups appear to have different norms? Did these differences help or hinder the groups in achieving their goals? Did some discussions or meetings proceed better than others? Why or why not? Rate the effectiveness of each group discussion or team meeting. Determine which behaviors appeared to help the most and the least, and identify areas for improvement.

CHAPTER 3

The Impact of Change on Teams and Teamwork

OBJECTIVES

After reading this chapter, you will be able to:

- *Compare traditional types of health care teams and today's new teams.*
- *Describe and give examples of self-directed, multifunctional, and transdisciplinary work teams.*
- *Define the term paradigm, and discuss why teams and teamwork represent the basis for a new paradigm in health care.*
- *Discuss the benefits of today's new teams from the employer, worker, and patient point of view.*

OVERVIEW

As might be expected, change has had, and is having, a tremendous impact on health care workers, teams, and teamwork. This chapter compares traditional teams with today's teams, and describes three types of new teams. Topics include how today's teams represent a new paradigm in health care, and their benefits.

As organizations restructure, redesign work, and cross-train employees, people often find themselves assigned to an on-going work team. Not only might they be working in a different area or in multiple areas performing a variety of functions, but also they are expected to work closely with others as a "well-oiled" team. This represents enormous change.

Traditionally, when workers participated as team members, they did so as specialists and as representatives of their respective disciplines. Their job titles and scopes of responsibilities were specific to their discipline. When they participated on teams, the teams themselves were somewhat loosely organized. An ample supply of supervisors and managers was usually on hand to establish and enforce policies, arrange schedules and work assignments, and help teams solve problems and achieve goals. That is not always the case today.

Teams have become an integral part of how health care organizations operate, and teams require more organization to function as smoothly as possible. Many workers now have team-based job titles and broader scopes of responsibility. Because of workforce downsizing, and the trend towards reducing layers of supervision and management, teams are expected to function with increasing independence, make higher level decisions, and solve more of their own problems.

SELF-DIRECTED WORK TEAMS

■ ***self-directed work teams:*** *groups with varying amounts of independence who have the authority to plan, conduct, evaluate, and control the work of the group*

Originating in manufacturing plants, **self-directed work teams** are becoming more common in today's health care organizations. Although levels of autonomy and responsibility vary, self-directed work teams often:

- develop their own work, holiday, and vacation schedules
- establish and monitor productivity and quality outcome goals
- develop budgets and allocate resources

- interview, select, orient, and train new team members
- assess and document team member competencies on an on-going basis
- conduct peer performance appraisals

MULTIFUNCTIONAL AND TRANSDISCIPLINARY TEAMS

■ ***paradigm:*** *a pattern or model*

■ ***multifunctional:*** *performing more than one function*

■ ***transdisciplinary:*** *across two or more disciplines*

Teams and teamwork represent the basis of a new **paradigm** in health care. Organizational restructuring, work redesign, multiskilling, and team-based care cause shifts in where employees work, what functions they perform, in which disciplines they work, and how they interact with one another. In restructured hospitals, where cross-training and team-based care have become prevalent, teams of multiskilled caregivers and support staff workers now provide up to 80 percent of all the services needed without patients having to leave their unit.

With job titles such as Team Care Member, Unit Representative, Service Associate, Unit Support Technician, Patient Care Assistant, Zone Service Worker, and Clinical Associate, these multiskilled workers serve on **multifunctional** or **transdisciplinary** teams. Because of the variety of job duties, they perform multiple functions, and their job responsibilities often span two or more different disciplines. Patient care assistants, for example, provide nursing, phlebotomy, and EKG functions, and unit support technicians have job duties in housekeeping, maintenance, and patient transportation.

In both inpatient and outpatient settings, increasing numbers of workers are now expected to cross-train and function as effective members of transdisciplinary teams. While caring for patients and providing high quality health services remain top priorities, how the work gets done may never be the same again.

> *"Twelve years ago when I started working at St. Vincent, we had to call different departments to do different things for our patients, like calling the lab to get blood work done. Back then, I worked as a team with an LPN. In some ways it was similar to how we work today. We checked with each other during the day to see how the other person was doing and to touch base on each of our patients. Today, the biggest change we've experienced with restructuring and multiskilling is that each of us has a broader role. For example, in the past we didn't have a tech on our unit who could do EKGs and phlebotomy for us, but now we do. In fact, we're all cross-trained to perform more functions, so any one of us could step up to the plate and do some of those extra things that none of us were used to doing in the past."*
>
> —JOAN BARR

BENEFITS OF TODAY'S TEAMS

Have these changes resulted in improvements? Many employers, employees, and patients would say "Yes!" Well functioning teams enhance communication, coordination, and continuity of care. Information is shared and work processes are streamlined. Decisions are made more quickly by those who work closely with the patients. Teams assigned to specific patients come to know their patients, and patients come to know their caregivers and support staff. Patient satisfaction and customer service increase, as does quality of care. Employers appreciate the increased flexibility, versatility, and productivity of the staff, and enhanced cost-effectiveness in the use of limited resources. Workers also report several benefits of being multiskilled team members. Job challenge increases as workers take on more responsibility. Team members have more input as to how things are done, and are able to see "the big picture" of what's going on with each patient. Self-esteem rises along with job satisfaction and job security. With cross-training and strong team skills, workers are more marketable, and enjoy enhanced opportunities for advancement.

> *"Working together to solve problems and knowing your input was heard makes you feel better about yourself in general . . . it's a more inclusive feeling. Having ownership of your job is a great feeling."*
>
> —Sammy Booker

Getting to the point where you are part of a smooth-running team is not easy. You will need to brush up on current skills and gain some new ones, and do not expect it to happen overnight.

Employers indicate that creating highly effective teams is one of their most difficult challenges. Doing so can take up to two years, in part because things keep changing so quickly in the health care field.

REVIEW QUESTIONS

1. Compare traditional types of health care teams with today's new teams.
2. Describe and give an example of a self-directed work team.
3. Which of the following are common activities of self-directed work teams? (Check all that apply)
   ____develop work, holiday, and vacation schedules
   ____provide supervision for other teams
   ____develop budgets and allocate resources
   ____orient new team members
   ____conduct peer performance appraisals
   ____establish pay rates for departmental staff
4. Define the terms multifunctional or transdisciplinary work teams, and give an example.
5. Give six benefits of today's new teams, listing two each from the employer, worker, and patient point of view.
6. Define the term paradigm.
7. Explain why today's teams represent a new paradigm in health care.

SUGGESTED LEARNING ACTIVITIES

1. Identify an organization that uses self-directed work teams. If possible, select a hospital or other type of health care organization. Invite one or more team members to meet with your class, or arrange a visit to the team's work place. Find out why the team was created, and determine its scope of responsibilities. Who serves on the team? How much autonomy and authority does the group have to make decisions? Is participating on a self-directed team different from working on a more traditional type of team? If so, how? What are the pro's and con's of serving on such a team? What challenges have the team encountered and how were they handled? What skills are needed to be effective? Where is the team headed in the future?
2. Interview members of a transdisciplinary or multifunctional team that works in a health care facility. If possible, interview patient caregivers, clerical workers, and support staff members. Find out why the team was created. Who serves on the team? What individual skills does each person bring to the team, and what are the team's overall scope of responsibilities? How does the team interact with other individuals and teams in the organization? How much autonomy and authority does the group have to make decisions?
3. Is participating on a transdisciplinary or multifunctional team different from working on a more traditional type of team? If so, how? What are the pro's and con's of serving on a team like this? What challenges has the team encountered and how were they handled? Are "turf" issues ever a problem? What skills are needed to be effective?
4. What benefits are derived from having these types of teams in the organization? How long did it take for the team to function smoothly? Where is the team headed in the future?
5. Form a team of classmates. Depending on how much responsibility and input to decision-making your instructor is willing to give the team, work together to identify:
   - course goals and objectives
   - course syllabus of topics
   - a schedule and location of class sessions
   - a list of guest speakers
   - potential field trips
   - criteria for determining final grades, if applicable.

   While working on this, remember the concept of group norms and the factors to be considered when evaluating team effectiveness. Consider videotaping your discussions to view later, and/or having someone in the group or an "outsider" volunteer to write down his or her observations and report them back to the group.

6. Form a team to help your supervisor with a project, such as revising a policy, setting up an inservice session, or arranging the work schedule for the next month. Depending on how much responsibility and input to decision-making your supervisor is willing to give the team, work together to identify:
   - goals and objectives of the project
   - a plan for organizing the project and completing it on time
   - a schedule and location for team meetings
   - a method for delegating responsibilities among individual team members
   - a list of necessary resources
   - periodic measurements to ensure the project is moving along as planned
   - criteria for evaluating outcomes to determine if the project was successful

   While working on this, remember the concept of group norms and the factors to be considered when evaluating team effectiveness. Consider videotaping your discussions to view later, and/or having someone in the group or an "outsider" volunteer to write down his or her observations and report them back to the group.

CHAPTER 4 What to Expect as a Health Care Team Member

OBJECTIVES

After reading this chapter, you will be able to:

- *Project the likelihood of becoming multiskilled and functioning in a team-based job.*
- *List and discuss six aspects of being a health care team member that you are likely to encounter.*
- *Explain why patients are increasingly viewed as members of the health care team.*
- *Discuss the impact of teamwork on individual performance appraisals and pay increases.*
- *Explain why new workers may have less difficulty than experienced workers participating in today's health care teams.*
- *Define and discuss occupational turf, matrix management, and peer pressure.*

OVERVIEW

This chapter describes what to expect as a health care team member, including the likelihood of becoming multiskilled and functioning in team-based jobs. It discusses patients as team members, the impact of teamwork on individual performance appraisals, and why new workers may have less difficulty participating on today's teams than more experienced workers. Topics include some of the challenges to be faced, including turf issues, matrix management, peer pressure, and changes in team membership.

Having realistic expectations is an important step in accomplishing your goals. Let us take a look at what you can expect in today's (and tomorrow's) health care workplace.

PARTICIPATION ON TEAMS

At some point in your career, it is likely that you will be cross-trained or retrained for a team-based job, and that your title and job description will reflect this. No matter where you work or what job you perform, expect to serve on many different teams during your career. Some will be the more traditional types of teams described earlier. Others will be the new kinds of teams currently evolving in redesigned workplaces. Some teams might even include patients as active team members. Today, consumers have more access to information on diseases, injuries, and treatment options than ever before. Patients ask more questions, and play a greater role in decision-making and their day-to-day health care.

Expect to be evaluated both for the contributions you make as an individual and those you make as a team member. Do not be surprised if your work performance is evaluated by the other members of your team, and if your pay raises are based, at least in part, on how well your team performs overall.

It is quite possible you may serve on more than one team at a time. Sometimes you will be a leader, other times a follower. Both are equally important and require special skills. Educators and employers can provide you with the training you need to perform the hands-on duties of your job, but finding workers with effective interpersonal skills is more difficult. Many times, managers say "Just give me a good team player and I'll take care of training them for job duties."

If you have been employed in a traditional health care job for some time, making the transition from functioning as an individual to working as a team member may be difficult. Being a team member requires different mind-sets as well as skills in negotiation, conflict resolution, and group dynamics. If you are starting your career, it may be easier for you than for existing workers, but you will need effective team skills.

> *"When we have a new RN join our patient-focused care unit that never knew the older way of doing things, it is no big deal. But for the older RN who always did the job one way, being cross-trained to perform additional tasks is not always appreciated. The benefit is being able to get the work done without having to call many different departments."*
>
> —JOAN BARR

CROSS-TRAINING

If you are used to functioning as a specialist, expect some challenges in cross-training. You may be asked to acquire additional skills, sometimes in disciplines other than the one you originally chose for your career. Do not view this expectation as abandoning your original occupation; instead, consider it an opportunity to expand your abilities and horizons. Explore some new ground and be willing to grow and learn new things.

■ ***occupational turf:*** *a set of functions or job responsibilities felt to be exclusive to workers in one discipline or occupational category*

If you are working in a newly redesigned department or patient care unit, and if you function as a multiskilled worker, you may encounter some **occupational turf** issues. Cross-training is still controversial among some individuals and groups of professionals who feel their exclusive territory is being invaded by others. Expect to have to prove yourself, especially if you are an extender. Make sure your job skills are up to the task, and demonstrate your abilities so that others can become familiar with them. It takes time to build trust and let others know you are reliable, especially when working in a job that is new to the organization.

SUPERVISION AND MANAGEMENT

Anticipate having to solve some problems yourself or within your team without expecting a supervisor or manager to step in and solve them for you. Depending on your job, you may be working with less direct supervision than has typically been the case in the past. As mentioned earlier, be sure you know the legal limitations of your responsibilities, and do not attempt to solve problems beyond that scope without appropriate help.

■ ***matrix management:*** *a situation where employees report to two or more managers from different departments or work units*

If you work on a multiskilled, transdisciplinary team, you may encounter situations where you report to more than one supervisor. Called **matrix management**, service associates working on patient care units, for example, might report to the nurse in charge of the unit as well as to a supervisor from environmental services or facilities management. Similarly, unit representatives might report to both a nursing unit manager and a supervisor in medical records or patient billing.

CHANGE AND CHALLENGES

Expect your role, and the role of your team, to constantly evolve over time. Team design is open to continual revision. Do not be surprised when things change and then change again.

You will likely encounter many challenges as you proceed. Just when your team begins to sail along smoothly, for example, someone will resign. Losing an experienced team member may cause a temporary setback, but if your team has a plan for orienting new members, you might gain some valuable new talent in the process.

■ ***peer pressure:*** *demands placed upon an individual by other workers of the same rank and status*

Peer pressure will be a major challenge. Expect it: it is how teams function. What happens when a team member does not do his or her share of the work, repeatedly fails to show up on time, or calls in sick too often? How will team members, including yourself, handle those situations? Upcoming chapters discuss skills that can help you meet these types of challenges.

> *"One of the biggest threats to the team is when someone isn't doing his or her share of the work. They sit back and wait for others to get the job done. But peer pressure usually takes care of the problem."*
>
> —Bonnie Hiner

REVIEW QUESTIONS

1. Discuss the likelihood of becoming multiskilled and functioning in a team-based job.
2. List and discuss six aspects of being a health care team member that you are likely to encounter.
3. Why are patients increasingly viewed as members of the health care team?
4. What impact does teamwork have on individual performance appraisals and pay increases?
5. Why might new workers may have less difficulty than experienced workers participating in today's health care teams?
6. Define and discuss occupational turf, matrix management, and peer pressure.

SUGGESTED LEARNING ACTIVITIES

1. Survey several personnel directors working in a variety of health care organizations and collect the following information:
   - Approximately what percent of workers were multiskilled ten years ago compared with the percent today, and what is the projected percentage five years from now?
   - Has cross-training created any professional turf issues? What are some examples?
   - To what extent are workers who have been retrained for jobs in greater demand?
   - What percent of workers currently function on teams? Is the number expected to increase over the next five years? Are self-directed work teams currently in use, and are they part of the plan for the future?
   - To what extent do patients participate as team members?
2. Recall a team experience you have had in your life. Were there any turf issues that arose? If so, what was the source of the problem, how did it challenge the group, and how was it handled? Was one or more members of the group ever queried about not doing his or her share of the work, or not following through with a responsibility? What was the source of the problem, how did it challenge the group, and how was it handled? Did peer pressure ever occur? What skills did you or other team members use to resolve turf issues or other problems that arose in the group?
3. Arrange an opportunity to serve on a project team. Examples might include setting up a health fair, career day, or web page for your school; undertaking a service project for your the community; or collaborating with co-workers on a quality improvement project. As the work of your team progresses, keep a record of each meeting and a personal log of observations. How well does the group work together? Are group norms evident? What role does each individual play? What characteristics and behaviors support or hinder the group's work? Do individual differences within the team help or pose challenges? How effective is the team? How effective are you as a team member? How could you and the team be more effective? Who is the leader of the team, and what leadership skills are evident?

CHAPTER 5 Skills for High Performance Work Teams

OBJECTIVES

After reading this chapter, you will be able to:

- *Define the terms functional and dysfunctional, and explain how they relate to the success of teams.*
- *List and discuss ten personal attributes and behaviors important in ensuring team success.*
- *Discuss the advantages of having different personality types on teams.*
- *Discuss the importance of knowing your job's parameters and legal scope of practice.*
- *Describe the value of accountability, life-long learning, managing stress and change, organizational and problem-solving skills, and interpersonal communication skills in teamwork.*
- *Define, give examples of, and compare aggressive, passive, passive-aggressive, and assertive communication styles.*
- *Define group dynamics, and explain how individual roles support or impede achieving consensus.*
- *Give five examples of cultural differences, and explain why diversity is important in health care teams.*
- *List four responsibilities of team leaders.*

OVERVIEW

This chapter discusses why some teams achieve success while others do not, and the wide variety of skills required to produce high-performance work teams. Topics include personal attributes, performing effectively within the scope of the job, and elements involved in group dynamics, valuing diversity, and leading teams.

Now that you are familiar with traditional and new types of teams in health care, and have a general idea of what to expect in the workplace, let us focus on what it takes to have an effective team.

Think back to some of the teams you have been part of in your life. Perhaps you played a team sport or worked with classmates on a school project. Maybe you joined a community organization and helped to plan a special event. Perhaps you served on a committee at work to review a procedure and recommend revisions. In any case, the experience of working with others to achieve a common goal has probably helped you realize it is not an easy process. Because you are part of a team and have a job to do does not necessarily mean the experience will be pleasant or successful. Many things can go wrong, impairing the team and rendering it unable to accomplish its goals. In fact, some teams are so **dysfunctional** it is a wonder they accomplish anything at all.

■ ***dysfunctional:*** *impaired; unable to achieve desired outcomes*

On the other hand, few things in life are more exhilarating than being part of a high-performance work team that is well-structured and able to meet, and

■ ***functional:*** *able to achieve desired outcomes*

even exceed, its goals. **Functional** teams can accomplish much more than any single individual, and the results are quite fulfilling. What has to happen to make sure your team is positioned for success?

SUCCESS BEGINS WITH YOU

Your team's success begins with you. A team is only as effective as each of its individual members. What are your own strengths, weaknesses, and areas for improvement? What special talents and characteristics do you bring to a team effort? Do you like working with people? If you consider yourself a "loner" and prefer working on your own, you should find a job that provides that kind of opportunity, or learn to enjoy working more closely with others.

■ ***self-discovery:*** *becoming aware of things about yourself that were previously unknown*

Spend some time on **self-discovery** to learn as much about yourself as possible. Book stores and libraries provide a wide variety of self-exploration and self-awareness resources, and school or career counselors can administer personal assessments to help you learn more about yourself than you ever knew before. Depending on the requirements of your job, you may need to "unlearn" some old behaviors and acquire new ones.

Several personal attributes will help guarantee your own success and that of your team. Are you honest, motivated, dependable, and reliable? Do you show initiative, accept responsibility, and follow through on commitments? Team members have to know they can count on each other.

Make sure you arrive for work on time every day, except when prevented from doing so by illness, injury, or emergency. When you get to your job site, show up ready to work. Remember that your patients always come first. Some days you may have to work through your lunch break, stay beyond regular work hours, or come in on your day off to provide coverage for a coworker. Whenever possible, volunteer to work a holiday that other team members need to have off, accept extra duties and work assignments, and be willing to help whenever and wherever you are needed. Making personal sacrifices on behalf of your patients and team members is an important part of being a health care professional.

Each team member has the power to make or break the team. Use this power wisely. Keep professional ethics in mind at all times. Apply the Golden Rule by treating others as you would want to be treated yourself. Keep private information in confidence, view your coworkers as "customers," and look for the good in people. Always give others the benefit of the doubt, do not spread gossip, and always be fair. Remember that individual competition is counterproductive to team work. Try to anticipate when a team member needs help, and be there to assist. Share information and resources, help coworkers learn and build confidence, and praise others for their accomplishments. When things go well, instead of boasting yourself, give your entire team the credit. When your team wins, you win.

Always strive to be part of the solution, not part of the problem. Keep a positive attitude, maintain your sense of humor, and never be afraid to laugh at yourself. These personal behaviors, and a commitment to your job, will serve you well and help forge strong relationships with your team members.

> *"The best team players are people who are self-motivated and career-minded; people who are willing to step up to the plate and accept responsibility. They're becoming harder to find."*
>
> —JOAN BARR

PERSONALITY TYPES

Wouldn't it be great if you could always choose your teammates? Unfortunately, in many situations, especially in jobs, you cannot. You must "take who you get" and make it work. There are many different personality types in our society: people with preferences like yours, and people who appear to be your exact opposites. Misunderstandings and disagreements among people with different personality types are frequent causes of friction. But the good news is, it takes all kinds of people to make effective teams. The challenge is knowing how best to use each person's unique characteristics.

■ ***complement:*** *two different parts that complete each other; something added to complete a whole*

Opposites **complement** each other. What would hot be without cold? What would sweet be without sour? What would Friday night be without Monday morning? One extreme to the other is what makes life interesting, and what helps teams get the job done. At first, you might think having team members with personalities like yours will make things easier. But consider the following examples. If you are an abstract thinker—a person who likes to dream and come up with "what ifs"—you enjoy the challenge of creating new ideas and innovative ways to approach things. Once the brainstorming is over, however, and a new approach is selected, you are ready to move on to the next "what if." But who is going to implement the new idea and see it through? Someone else on your team might be less of an abstract thinker and more of a "here and now" type person. He or she may not enjoy the brainstorming phase, but like implementing new ideas once they have been identified. Although different, your two personality types complement one another, and both are necessary to see a project through from beginning to end.

■ ***introvert:*** *a person whose thoughts and attentions are drawn inward, within him or herself*

■ ***extrovert:*** *a person whose thoughts and attentions are turned outward, towards other people*

Perhaps you are an **introvert**, a person who likes to work quietly behind the scenes. When your team is asked to analyze some financial data and present the results, the analysis may sound good to you, but presenting the report in front of a group might not. An **extrovert** on your team, however, may dislike delving into data but enjoy public speaking. Again, because your personality types complement one another, both of you can work together to achieve success and enjoy the roles each of you played.

Teams benefit from a variety of personality types. The challenge is to know each other's personalities and preferences well enough to determine how to make the best use of individual differences. Not only will the team be more successful in reaching its goals, but also the members will have more fun doing something they enjoy and at which they are good.

What is your personality type? There are several different kinds of questionnaires and "tools" to help you learn more about your personality preferences. One of the best known is the Myers-Briggs Type Indicator (MBTI). The MBTI has been in use for more than 50 years, and validated many times for its accuracy. By completing a simple questionnaire, your results place you in one of 16 different personality types. Knowing your type, and those of your teammates, can help members understand what makes them similar to, or different from, the others on the team. Armed with this valuable information, teams can make better decisions dividing up work tasks and meeting tough challenges.

INTERPERSONAL RELATIONSHIPS AND SHARED MISSION

Establishing good interpersonal relationships is one of the best ways to strengthen teamwork and learn more about the personalities and preferences of your teammates. Spend some time with coworkers during lunch breaks or after hours, and volunteer for special projects to get to know each person as an individual and to help others get to know you better. Do your part to cultivate a team spirit and a sense of shared purpose. After all, everyone's mission at work is the same: to care for patients and provide quality health services for people who need them. When the going gets rough, always keep that shared mission in mind.

> *"If there's a common goal for the team, a common focus, it is amazing how quickly and how well the job can get done. Just think how well people pull together in a disaster situation."*
>
> —Diana Graham

Teams need a clear understanding of their goals, objectives, expectations, and the criteria by which their success will be measured. They also need to know how much autonomy or independence they have and to what extent they are permitted to make decisions without additional approval. Make sure you understand these **parameters** yourself, and are familiar with all of the policies and procedures that govern your workplace.

■ ***parameters:*** *boundaries, limits, scopes of responsibility*

ROLE CLARIFICATION AND LEGAL ISSUES

Team members also need a clear understanding of individual roles and responsibilities and how work is supervised and delegated. These are important issues for every team, but especially for transdisciplinary and multifunctional work teams. These kinds of teams require extra coordination because of the diversity in skills and functions performed. How does your team fit into the "big picture" of caring for patients and providing health-related services? How does your team interact with other individuals and other teams?

In today's restructured organizations, it might take some time for you to fully understand your role and to accept it. It also takes time for coworkers to fully understand and value each other's roles and abilities. As mentioned earlier, teams of patient caregivers must be familiar with each other's abilities so they know who they can trust to perform certain functions, especially in emergency situations. Caregivers must also understand the roles of support teams and clerical teams, and how all of the different groups interact and depend on one another to get work done. If you are unsure about the roles, responsibilities, and relationships among the different teams where you work, ask for clarification. When a new team member joins your work group, be sure the person is well oriented to his or her role, and understands the interconnectedness of the other teams.

Legal scopes of practice may also come into play, especially for patient caregivers. For example, nurse extenders (patient care technicians and patient care assistants) work under the direct supervision of registered nurses, and have legal limitations as to what they can do. Because health care workers are especially vulnerable to legal action, it is absolutely vital that each team member be familiar with these limitations and that workers function within legal boundaries. If you ever have *any* questions about what you can and cannot do legally, be sure to ask a supervisor or manager for clarification. Know your limits and ask for help when you need it. Operating outside your legal scope of practice puts you, your patients, coworkers, and employer at risk.

When you think of delegating work, you probably think of a higher-skilled person or a supervisor delegating tasks to a lower-skilled, nonsupervisory worker. While this is often the case, the opposite is sometimes true also. On a patient care unit, for example, registered nurses are responsible for patient assessment. A nurse may delegate taking a patient's blood pressure to a competent patient care technician (PCT). But when the PCT notices something abnormal about the patient, he or she delegates responsibility back to the nurse who checks on the patient. In order for teams to function effectively, members must understand their roles in delegating work and having work delegated to them. It all comes back to role clarification, and safely operating within one's job description and legal scope of practice.

> *"When everyone understands what part they play, things go much smoother"*
>
> —BONNIE HINER

ACCOUNTABILITY

Even when each person's role and responsibilities are clear, things can still go wrong. Consider the following.

> *This is a story about four people: everybody, somebody, anybody, and nobody. There was an important job to be done and everybody was sure somebody would do it. Anybody could do it, but nobody did it. Somebody got angry about that, because it was everybody's job. Everybody thought anybody could do it. But nobody realized that everybody wouldn't do it. It ended up that everybody blamed somebody when nobody did what anybody could have done.*
>
> —AUTHOR UNKNOWN

Coordinating team efforts to make sure that everything gets done, and done well, is a major challenge, one you are likely to face every day on the job. Do not just assume someone else will complete the task: *make sure* it gets done. If one person fails, the team fails. Saying "That's not my job" is unacceptable. Even if *doing* the job is not part of your responsibility, *making sure* the information is communicated to the right person is.

ORGANIZATIONAL AND PROBLEM SOLVING SKILLS

A primary benefit of teamwork is getting the work done more efficiently. This requires good organizational and problem-solving skills, as well as the ability to establish priorities. Did you ever miss appointments because you forgot them? Did you ever start projects and later realize you did not have the supplies you needed to complete them? Dis you ever miss deadlines because you did not start soon enough, or got bogged down trying to make decisions? Did you ever have trouble deciding where to start?

Planning ahead, being organized, and solving problems are all crucial elements of success, both for individuals and for team members. Learn how to establish priorities and manage your time effectively. What needs to be done first? In what order do tasks need to be accomplished? How much time needs to be allocated for each step in the process? What outcome must be achieved before moving on to the next step? How should your workspace be set up to facilitate productivity? How do tasks and assignments need to be delegated and coordinated to ensure all steps in the process are completed correctly and on time?

A major barrier to achieving goals is a disorganized approach to work. Organize your thoughts in advance, and communicate with others on a regular basis. Coordinate your efforts with coworkers to be certain everyone is moving in the right direction and on schedule. Allow extra time for preparation, and avoid overextending yourself. Keep a pocket-sized calendar with you at all times, and enter your work schedule, meetings, appointments, family plans, social outings, and special events. Note deadlines, bill payment dates, and other information. When you have a project coming up, determine when you need to get started and note that date on your calendar. Refer to your calendar frequently, and make sure it is up to date.

■ ***proactive:*** *to take action in advance, before the need occurs*

■ ***reactive:*** *to respond and take action after a need has occurred*

Be **proactive** rather than **reactive**. Think, plan ahead, and anticipate needs before they occur. Make sure your work area is well stocked with the tools and supplies you need, and keep it neat and orderly. If you are responsible for maintaining requisitions, records, or other kinds of paperwork, set up a good filing system and use it. Make sure coworkers know where you keep things in case something has to be retrieved in your absence.

Learn to solve problems efficiently and creatively. Get to the root of the problem and determine optimal outcomes. If the problem seems too complex, break it down into smaller, more solvable pieces. Identify your options, assess the pro's and con's of each, weigh in factors such as urgency and potential risk, and develop a plan for arriving at a solution. Stay focused, be aware of time constraints, and the affect your decisions may have on others.

Be open to new ways of addressing old problems. As a health care worker, you will be challenged to "think outside the box." Develop good critical thinking skills and apply them. A new twist on an old approach might be just the answer you are looking for.

MANAGING STRESS AND CHANGE

Working in health care can be stressful, especially today with so much change occurring all around you. When the impact of change adds to the pressures of working in a team-based job, you may have to find ways to help alleviate your stress and protect your health. Talking with others who understand your feelings can be extremely therapeutic. Participating in a support group might help, especially if you work with sick children or terminally ill patients. Team members can help each other deal with death and dying, and provide other types of emotional support when needed. All too often, caregivers devote so much time and energy taking care of others, they neglect themselves. Do everything you can to help manage your own stress and that of your teammates.

A few years ago, health care workers needed skills to *cope* with change. But now, rapid change is such a common part of our jobs that coping is not enough anymore. To be truly effective in today's environment, you need to *adapt* to change, *embrace* it, and perhaps even *lead* change. How you handle change may need more consideration. If you are the type of person who dislikes change and functions best in a stable, predictable environment, working in today's health care system could be especially stressful. Keep in mind that while change can be upsetting and produce anxiety, it also can lead to improvements and new opportunities.

The teams on which you participate will experience many changes, not the least of which is losing experienced members and gaining new ones. Change in membership is one of the most stressful events than can happen to a team. Think back to what it was like when you first joined the group. Do whatever you can to help new people feel welcome. Remember, new team members are in the midst of stressful change, too.

LIFE-LONG LEARNING

The most vital contributions you bring to the team are your knowledge, skills, and abilities. Keep your skills up to date, and never stop learning. Learn from your mistakes, seize new opportunities for growth, continually strive for quality, and make a commitment to getting better every day at what you do.

INTERPERSONAL COMMUNICATION SKILLS

Effective communication is a major key to success in daily living and in just about every kind of job and workplace. Rarely does a day go by when you will not be challenged by the need to give and receive information through interactions with a variety of people. Poor communication is the leading cause of interpersonal conflict, misunderstandings, disagreements, arguments, and confrontations with others. Strong interpersonal communication skills give you the tools you need to resolve those kinds of conflicts.

As might be expected, effective communication skills are absolutely vital for health care workers, especially those working on teams. How effective a communicator are you? Are you good at getting your point across to others? Can you disagree with someone but still demonstrate respect for his or her opinions? Can you offer constructive criticism without hurting another person's feelings? How sharp are your listening skills? Do you try to understand the other person's point of view even when it is different from your own?

Let us examine a common, conflict-causing situation, and test some different communication styles to determine which one works best. Two cars, one driven by a man and the other by a woman, pull up to a four-way stop, proceed through the intersection at the same time, and collide. Both drivers leap out of their cars and confront each other face-to-face. Four different communication styles could emerge.

1. The man, angry because his car has been damaged, verbally attacks the woman. "You idiot! Why don't you learn to drive?" he shouts. "Me?" the woman exclaims, "you are the one who ran the stop sign. Are you blind?"

   Aggressive communication rarely resolves conflicts because a personal, verbal attack makes the other person angry and defensive. Because neither the man nor the woman showed any respect for each other, the situation can only get worse.

■ ***aggressive communication:*** *bold and domineering; disrespectful of the opinions and feelings of others*

2. The same verbal attack occurs, but this time the woman replies meekly, "I'm so sorry. I'm sure this was all my fault. I just can't seem to do anything right. When my husband finds out, he's going to be furious!"

   Passive communication leaves the man feeling smug (although the collision might actually have been his fault), and the woman looking and feeling like a floor mat.

■ ***passive communication:*** *stating no opposition, submissive; devaluing one's own opinion and feelings*

3. The same verbal attack occurs, and the same meek-appearing woman claims it must have been all her fault. But as the man smugly walks back to his car, the woman secretly stabs one of his rear tires with a sharp, metal nail file she keeps in her purse.

   Passive-aggressive communication is not the answer either. Although the woman may feel vindicated for having "gotten even" with the man, she did so in a cowardly and illegal way.

■ ***passive-aggressive communication:*** *appearing submissive but underhandedly aggressive; dishonest and disrespectful*

4. When the man verbally attacks the woman, she ignores his personal comments and calmly responds, "Since we both arrived at a four-way stop at the same time, and I was to your right, I believe I had the right of way. I'll phone the police department, and when the officer arrives we will ask for clarification. If we still disagree, our insurance companies can decide who's legally at fault. In any case, this is certainly an unfortunate situation for both of us."

   Assertive communication allows the woman to state her own view of what happened without attacking the man. Assertive communication is usually the most effective way to resolve interpersonal conflict.

■ ***assertive communication:*** *a positive and confident statement of opinion; respectful of all points of view*

What if a similar situation had occurred in the workplace?

In the first scenario, workers who allow their conflict to escalate into aggressive behavior will likely face disciplinary action and possible termination. Aggressive communication rarely has a place in the workplace. In the second scenario, passive communication is no solution either. Health care workers must have sufficient self-esteem and courage to stand up for themselves and not allow others to walk all over them. Passive people are viewed as pitiful, which is definitely not a desirable trait. The passive-aggressive communication in the third scenario is even worse, representing totally unacceptable behavior and grounds for disciplinary action or termination.

The assertive communication displayed by the woman in the fourth and final scenario is the preferred style, both on the job and in other aspects of life. You must be able to state your opinions openly and honestly while still treating the other person and their feelings with respect. Assertive communication is not easy. You must control your own anger while overlooking the aggressive behavior of the other person. It takes courage and practice to communicate assertively. If this is a problem for you, take a course in assertive communication. You may need to unlearn some old behaviors and replace them with new, more effective behaviors.

Now that you are familiar with these four styles of communication, watch how other people use them, and observe the kinds of responses they get. Watch what happens when two people get angry with one another and resort to personal attacks. Observe passive and passive-aggressive behaviors to see what happens. Then watch assertive communicators and learn from their experiences. With sufficient observation, you will soon realize that assertive communication offers the best chance for a win-win situation.

Now it is your turn. Although it might feel uncomfortable, it is your responsibility to speak up when you disagree with someone or something. Your employer did not hire you to be a mindless puppet. You are there to contribute to the organization's mission which sometimes means disagreeing with someone or going against popular opinion. This is not to say you should fight every battle that presents itself. Remember the old saying "Choose your battles carefully." If it is a minor disagreement with no major ramifications, perhaps it is best to let it go. But if you think your patients or coworkers might be at risk, or if for any other reason you feel it is in the best interests of those you serve, speak up and make your concerns known.

If you are not used to standing up for yourself with family members or in social settings, expect it to be equally difficult at work. Experiment by starting with a low-risk situation (do not experiment on your spouse or your boss). Consider confronting someone who steps in front of you in line, send your meal back when it is not what you ordered, or question the extra charge on a bill. When confronting someone, make eye contact and keep your voice level, steady, and calm. If the other person is standing, you should stand as well. If this is a totally new kind of communication style for you, expect to be a little shaky the first few times you try being assertive. Consider sweaty palms a sign of personal growth!

> *"Developing effective team skills takes time because you are asking people to change behaviors. If you are a person who's used to being submissive at home, it is hard to learn to confront coworkers on the job"*
>
> —Rita Emerick

Just because you think you have handled a situation appropriately, do not assume the other person is automatically going to fall into line. The important thing is to use good assertive communication skills yourself, and do the best you can to resolve the conflict. Although your own actions may influence the reactions of others, accept the fact that you cannot control someone else's behavior.

No discussion about effective communication would be complete without addressing the need for good listening skills. Communication is a two-way process. Understanding what the other person is saying is just as important as stating your own message effectively. Always concentrate when listening, and repeat the message back in your own words to make sure your understanding is accurate. If you want people to listen to you and understand what you have to say, you must listen to them and understand their message. Active listening shows respect for the other person, and can help prevent misunderstandings that often lead to conflict.

■ ***body language:*** *nonverbal communication characterized by posture, eye-contact, facial expressions, etc.*

Not all communication is verbal. Learn to observe **body language** and other nonverbal cues. You can tell a lot about how someone feels by their facial expressions and gestures, how they sit or stand, and whether or not they make eye contact with you.

If your job requires dealing face-to-face with angry people on a regular basis, consider some additional training in how to de-escalate difficult situations. Angry, loud people may become abusive and violent. Special skills are needed to protect yourself and manage those kinds of conflicts.

Giving constructive criticism without hurting a person's feelings calls for advanced communication skills. Go back to the Golden Rule. If someone was to critique your performance, how would you want him or her to do it? As mentioned previously, some types of work teams use peer performance appraisals. You will be evaluating the work of your teammates, and they will be evaluating yours. Talk about stress! When appraising your teammate's performance, identify as many positives as you can, and communicate the negatives in a constructive, supportive manner. Offer help and concrete suggestions for improvement. When your own performance is being appraised by someone else, use your listening skills to avoid misunderstandings. Be open-minded, try to see things from the other person's perspective, and do not jump to conclusions. Accept the fact that no one is perfect. If you avoid becoming defensive and really listen, you might gain some valuable feedback.

> *"Sometimes there's a need to defend yourself, your point of view. As a team, we had to learn to do that without hurting another person's feelings."*
>
> —NEDDA GRIFFEN

Even if you do not work on a team that does peer performance appraisals, you still may need to give coworkers feedback about their work. If you must be critical of someone's performance, your first inclination might be to report your concerns to the person's supervisor and let them worry about it. Doing so, however, is taking the easy way out. If someone had a complaint about you, would you prefer they discuss it with you first or go directly to your supervisor? If you do take the situation to a supervisor, his or her first question will likely be, "Have you tried discussing this problem with your coworker yourself?" If a teammate is not pulling his or her share of the load, or if weak performance or unethical behaviors are undermining the organization's efforts, go directly to the person in question and address the situation head-on. Your coworker will probably respect you for it. Use your assertive communication and active listening stills, and be as positive and supportive as possible. Do not procrastinate. The problem will only get worse as your anxiety level gets higher.

Being on a team provides ample opportunity to work on your communication and listening skills. Learn as much as you can about effective communication, and practice, practice, practice. There is always room for improvement.

GROUP DYNAMICS AND CONSENSUS

■ ***group dynamics:*** *tensions, interrelationships, and interactions between two or more people in a group setting*

Understanding **group dynamics** and the different "roles" people play within groups is of great importance when working with teams, and especially during team meetings.

Let us start with you. What role do you usually play in group settings? Are you the quiet one that rarely says anything unless pressured to do so? Do you dominate the discussion, interrupting other people every time you have something to say yourself? Do you play "the devil's advocate," always critiquing other people's suggestions and questioning their input?

The roles we play in groups are often connected with our individual personality types. Someone who scores high on the introvert scale, for example, may not volunteer much input in a group setting unless they are asked to or concerned that the group is headed in the wrong direction. Extroverts, on the other hand, may be more comfortable in a group setting, and lead the discussion. Other personality characteristics become apparent in group settings. "Harmonizers" try to keep everyone happy and make sure all opinions get voiced. "Clarifiers" restate what others have said to be certain everyone's clear on the message. "Diagnosers" identify barriers keeping the group from achieving its goals. "Clowns" joke around and distract the group from its work. "Blockers" impede process. "Consensus builders" poll group members to help them reach an agreement.

People do not always play the same role in different groups and in different settings. It often comes down to comfort levels and acceptance or nonacceptance by other group members. In a family situation, for example, a woman might take the lead in deciding how to invest some extra income. But at work, she might defer financial decisions to the men in the group. An introvert may have little to say in a group overrun with vocal "dominators." But in a different group, where each person's opinion is valued, he or she might participate more fully. A "harmonizer" might thrive in one group where relationships are important, but be shut down by "blockers" in a different group.

Understanding group dynamics comes with experience. Observing the roles played by others, and the impact they have, will help you learn what works and what does not work. Holding your own in a group depends on your interpersonal communication skills. Using assertive communication skills gives you the opportunity to be heard while respecting everyone else's opinions. There is no doubt that a single person can shut down the entire group process. If that happens in your group, you may need to confront the offender or work with other members to remove that person from the group.

To be an effective group member, you will need to be a full participant. Playing a certain role is acceptable as long as it is productive, and supports meeting goals and objectives. Help the group stay focused, encourage and support each member's participation, willingly provide information, contribute ideas and options, and be open-minded and willing to compromise.

If you have the opportunity to help form a group and select its members, consider including people with different personality types. Remember that opposites complement one another. The dynamics of a group composed of different personalities will create more challenges, but sound decisions and successful outcomes emanate from a variety of perspectives. If everyone in the group thinks the same way you do, something important might be overlooked.

■ ***consensus:*** *an agreement acceptable to everyone*

Negotiating skills are very helpful in group dynamics. The goal is to identify each person's individual position on the topic at hand, and then find "common ground" acceptable to all members. Achieving **consensus** does not necessarily mean there is a unanimous vote, or that the agreed-upon outcome is each person's first choice. Consensus simply means that each member of the group can live with the decision and support it. In consensus, there are no losers. Each group member must be flexible, open to other people's opinions, and willing to compromise. Achieving consensus is not always possible, and sometimes group members have to just "agree to disagree."

VALUING DIVERSITY

■ ***cultural differences:*** *factors such as age, gender, race, ethnic heritage, lifestyle preference, socioeconomic status, occupational classification, and physical condition*

Much has already been said about different personality types, and the roles that such differences play in teamwork. But in working with a variety of people, you also encounter many **cultural differences**, based on factors such as age, gender, race, ethnic heritage, lifestyle preference, socioeconomic status, occupational classification, and physical condition. There is no question that cultural differences can sometimes create difficult challenges, but they often bring a variety of perspectives to the situation, and add the richness of diversity.

Americans live in a multicultural society, and it is important to understand diversity and become comfortable with it. Years ago, when interest in diversity issues heightened, people were encouraged to *tolerate* differences. But today, a greater percentage of our population has come to *value* diversity, and apply its strengths to benefit everyone.

Cultural differences affect people's values and the way they approach life and work. To best work with people from different cultures, it helps to "walk in their shoes" and view life from their perspective. Let people get to know you, your background, values, and cultural traits better. Learn as much as you can about diversity, and discuss cultural differences with coworkers and friends. Attend churches other than your own, participate in multicultural events, read up on age- and gender-specific characteristics, spend time with the physically challenged, and shadow workers in other disciplines.

Diversity issues are often at the forefront in health care as you encounter people from all walks of life. Some represent races, foreign nationalities, and age groups different from your own. Some are wealthy, and others barely make ends meet. Some are young, others older. Some prescribe patient treatments whereas others mop floors, prepare meal trays, or repair malfunctioning equipment. Each person plays an important role, but few can attain success without the efforts of others. Regardless of whether you are a nurse, technologist, therapist, clerical worker or support staff member, everyone shares the common mission of providing high-quality health care services. Taking care of patients and other customers provides more than ample common ground to overcome divisiveness.

Issues related to personal values present some of the toughest diversity challenges. Based on your cultural background and life experiences, you may have some strong feelings about things such as abortion, assisted suicide, genetic cloning, gay rights, and prayer in school. In a democracy such as ours, there is no right or wrong when it comes to personal values and cultural perspectives. Each person has a constitutional right to his or her own beliefs. Just as you expect others to respect your values and your beliefs, you must respect the values and beliefs of others. This is not to say you must *agree* with, or *condone*, a point of view radically different from your own; but only that you try to *accept* these differences and learn to function in spite of them.

Our nation still has a long way to go in accepting cultural differences. But a team of health care workers striving to better understand one another, and work together for the common good of their patients, represents a big step forward.

LEADERSHIP

As mentioned earlier, sometimes you will be expected to play the role of a leader, and at other times, that of a follower. Both are important roles and require some special skills.

Shared leadership is becoming more common in health care today. As a team member, you may have the opportunity to lead your team. Being a team leader is not the same as being a supervisor. Supervisors have workers who report to them, and the supervisor is held accountable for the work of subordinates. Team leaders, on the other hand, do not have "direct reports" and are not held personally accountable for the performance of their teammates.

Several functions of supervisors and team leaders do overlap, however, and both need similar skills. Like supervisors, team leaders serve as facilitators and coaches. They organize and coordinate activities, line up resources, monitor the efforts of coworkers, track progress, and report results. Team leaders help solve problems, and make sure everyone has input into decisions and access to the latest information. They identify staff development and training needs and arrange continuing education sessions, lead team meetings, and help manage group dynamics.

Being the leader of a team is a great opportunity for you to practice what you have learned, and to acquire some new and valuable skills. Unfortunately, it is not unusual to be thrust into a leadership role without extra training to help you be more successful. If this happens to you, take the initiative to sign up for some special classes, and do some additional reading to prepare for your new responsibilities. Work closely with your supervisor so you know exactly what is expected of you, and ask your supervisor and coworkers for regular feedback regarding your performance. Becoming an effective leader takes time and commitment, but the extra effort can lead to new opportunities for those who develop effective leadership skills.

Being an effective follower also requires skills and commitment. Accepting assignments, following directions, communicating and cooperating with others, and completing tasks on time are all vital elements to achieving success. If one person "drops the ball" by failing to complete his or her task or assignment appropriately and on time, the work of the entire group may be jeopardized. High-performance work teams require strong leaders and strong followers.

SUMMARY

No one can wave a magic wand and produce high-performance work teams. Effective teams and team members are the product of hard work, commitment, time, patience, and practice. Each individual must play his or her role in helping the team achieve success. Whether you participate on a daily basis as a work team member with one or several other people, or serve on project teams to improve patient care and services, the role you play is critical to the success of your organization.

Developing effective team skills is an on-going process, and well worth the effort. You will always have new challenges to tackle, and more things to learn. But what is most important is that you are well prepared and committed to always doing your best. Your patients and teammates deserve it, and so do you.

REVIEW QUESTIONS

1. Define the terms functional and dysfunctional, and explain how they relate to the success of teams.
2. List ten personal attributes and behaviors important in ensuring team success.
3. Discuss the advantages of having different personality types on teams.
4. Why is it important to know your job's parameters and legal scope of practice?
5. Describe accountability and explain its importance in teamwork.
6. What does life-long learning mean, and why is it important for health care workers?
7. List two sources of job-related stress, and explain the importance of team members having stress management skills.
8. What is the difference between coping with change and embracing change?
9. Explain the difference between being proactive and reactive, and indicate which is best, and why.
10. Explain the value of having good organizational and problem-solving skills
11. Define interpersonal communication and discuss its role in teamwork.
12. Why are good listening skills and awareness of body language important in teamwork?
13. Describe the following interpersonal communication styles, and give an example of each: aggressive, passive, passive-aggressive, and assertive.
14. Of the four interpersonal communication styles, which one is best, and why?
15. Define the terms group dynamics and consensus.
16. List four different roles commonly seen in group dynamics, and explain how each role either supports or impedes achieving consensus.
17. List five examples of cultural differences.
18. Discuss tolerating and valuing diversity.
19. Discuss the potential challenges and benefits of having diversity within a health care team.
20. List four responsibilities of team leaders, and compare the roles of team leaders and supervisors. List four responsibilities of followers, and explain why being an effective follower is as important as being an effective leader.

SUGGESTED LEARNING ACTIVITIES

1. Observe a health care team in action in the workplace and record what you notice. What were the goals of the team? How well did team members work together? Were group norms evident? Was each team member's role clear? Rate the effectiveness of the team using factors identified earlier. List some examples of what worked well and what did not work well, and explain why. What individual skills did you observe? What group or team skills were evident? Were these skills effective? Did team members display good organizational and problem solving skills? Was accountability evident? What do you think would help the team function better? If you were part of this team, how would you help team members achieve their goals?
2. Sit in on a group meeting and record what you observe. What was the purpose of the meeting? Describe the composition of the group. Could you tell why each person had been asked to participate? How well did the group work together? What styles of interpersonal communication were used? Did individuals listen to one another and respect different opinions? What body language did you observe? Were different personality types evident? If so, describe the different types and how well they interacted. Was diversity within the group evident? If so, describe the diversity, and discuss its impact on group dynamics. What roles did individual group members play? Did these roles enhance or impede the group's work? Who was the leader of

the group? What leadership skills were displayed and how effective were they? Did the group need to achieve consensus? If so, what steps were taken? Were they successful? If you were a member of this group, what would you do to help the group achieve its goals?

3. Observe three different interpersonal confrontations and record what happened. What caused each confrontation and who was involved? What styles of interpersonal communication were evident, and how well did each work in resolving the conflict? Were the parties involved listening to one another? Were they displaying respect for one another? If you had been involved in each of these confrontations yourself, how would you have handled the situation?
4. Set up some role-playing scenarios involving confrontations between two people. Using each of the four different styles of interpersonal communication, try to resolve the conflict. Which communication style feels the most comfortable to you? Which seems to work best, and why?
5. Select a controversial ethical or legal issue where people might have opposite points of view. Some examples are assisted suicide, right-to-life, and cloning. Set up a discussion or debate, and give each person the opportunity to state his or her opinion. During the discussion, if people interrupt one another, or if more than one person tries to speak at once, use a "talking stick." The talking stick is some object that an individual must have in his or her possession before being allowed to speak. Only the person with the talking stick may speak, and while doing so, others in the group must listen. When the speaker has finished, the talking stick is passed on to someone else, and that person then has the floor. At the conclusion of the discussion, describe what happened. Did values and cultural differences influence individual points of view? If so, how? Were participants given ample opportunity to be heard, or was the talking stick necessary? How well did you use your listening skills? Did you fully understand points of view different from your own? Did you feel listened to and understood yourself? Was mutual respect among participants evident? How can you apply what was learned from this experience in your work as a team member?
6. Determine your own personality type by working with a school counselor or vocational advisor who can administer an assessment for you. Describe the characteristics of your personality type. How does your personality type compare or differ from others? What unique challenges might you face based on your type? What personality type would be the opposite of yours? If you worked with someone whose type was opposite from yours, what challenges would both of you likely face? What personality types would complement your own? If possible, have coworkers, family members, or school mates also take the personality assessment. How do their types compare with yours? Does awareness of these different types help explain how well you do, or do not, interact with those around you? How can you use this knowledge to improve teamwork and interpersonal communication?
7. Identify a project you need to complete. Before beginning the project, make a list of the different steps in the process, determine what should happen first, and organize the remaining steps according to the sequence in which they need to occur. Develop an overall schedule to finish the project on time, and note a deadline for completing each of the steps along the way. As you work through the project, keep a written log to record what you did and when you did it. After the project has been completed, compare your written log with the schedule you originally developed. Did establishing priorities, setting deadlines, and organizing your approach in advance help you accomplish your goal on time? What organizational and time-management skills did you learn through this process, and how can these skills be applied to future projects and team efforts?
8. Using this chapter as a reference, compile a list of skills necessary to function as an effective team member. Use the list to determine which skills you already possess and which ones you need to improve. Develop a personal improvement plan for those skills that require some additional work. List specific goals, steps needed to accomplish each goal, and a time schedule for completing your personal improvement plan. As you proceed, ask people for feedback, note your progress, and practice your new skills. Repeat this process of self-inventory and personal improvement on a regular basis.
9. As a group activity, identify several people that group members know, or have observed in action, who demonstrate strong leadership skills. Make a list of the characteristics and behaviors that contribute to the success of these leaders. Add any additional characteristics or behaviors that you and your group members think are important when participating in team activities. Use this list to develop a rating system to evaluate the effectiveness of yourself and others when serving in a leadership capacity.
10. If you have videotapes of group discussions or team meetings, view the tapes again, and watch for different characteristics and behaviors of people who assumed leadership roles. Observe what did and did not work well, and why, and evaluate the leaders' effectiveness. What opportunities for improvement can be identified? Plan a team activity and allow each member to serve in a leadership role sometime during the course of the project. Encourage each person to remember the characteristics and behaviors of effective leaders that were identified earlier. Help each team member evaluate his or her effectiveness by offering constructive feedback, and work toward improving leadership skills by gaining more and more experience.

SUPPLEMENTAL RESOURCES

Games Teams Play: Dynamic Activities for Tapping Work Team Potential

A "team development system" of 52 games, activities, and "workouts," to help develop new teams and strengthen existing ones. Uses team development activities as catalysts to promote team growth. Includes reproducible handouts. 1996. By Leslie Bendaly,
McGraw-Hill Ryerson Limited
300 Water Street
Whitby, Ontario L1N 9B6

Ordering information:
McGraw-Hill Priority Processing
P.O. Box 182605
Columbus, OH 43272-3032
1-800-2-MCGRAW
614-759-3644 (Fax)
ISBN 0-07-552718-9 (paperback) or 0-07-552719-7 (looseleaf)

Subarctic Survival Situation

A survival scenario involving the crash-landing of an airplane in a subarctic region of Canada, where passengers must work as individuals and team members to overcome the life-threatening challenges they face. 1987 By J. Clayton Lafferty, Ph.D.
Human Synergistics International
39819 Plymouth Road C-8020
Plymouth, MI 48170
1-800-622-7584 or 734-459-1030
734-459-5557 (Fax)

Self-Managed Work Teams in Health Care Organizations

Written for TQM/CQI programs and patient-centered care hospitals, this 264-page book discusses the advantages of self-managed work teams, team design and development, compensation and rewards, and making teams work. By Elizabeth D. Becker-Reems.
American Hospital Publishing, Inc. (an American Hospital Association Company)
AHA Services, Inc.
P.O. Box 92683
Chicago, IL 60675-2683
1-800-AHA-2626
312-280-6015 (Fax)
Catalogue number B43-169109

It's a Jungle Out There! An Insider's Outlook on Jobs in Health Care

Written for students, teachers, advisors, and parents, this up-to-date booklet describes why and how health care is changing, and the impact of change on career and employment opportunities. Discusses organizational restructuring, work redesign, multiskilling, and new roles for health care workers. Topics include the role of teams, skills in demand, and how to prepare for the health care workplace of tomorrow. 1996 By Sherry Makely, Ph.D., RT(R)
Pine Ridge Publications, Inc.
1051 West Burma Road
Bloomington, IN, 47404
812-876-7211
812-876-9117 (Fax)
ISBN 0-9652954-0-0

Multiskilled Health Care Workers: Issues and Approaches to Cross-Training

Written for managers, educators, workers, and students, this book describes the evolution of cross-training, and how multiskilled personnel provide team-based care in today's restructured health care organizations. Topics include skill combinations, team composition, and approaches to educating and employing multiskilled personnel. 1998 By Sherry Makely, Ph.D., RT(R)

Pine Ridge Publications, Inc.
1051 West Burma Road
Bloomington, IN, 47404
phone 812-876-7211
812-876-9117 (Fax)
ISBN 0-9652954-3-5

Introduction to Type in Organizations

Examines applications of the Myers-Briggs Type Indicator (MBTI) in the workplace. Second Edition by Sandra Krebs Hirsh and Jean M. Kummerow.

Consulting Psychologists Press, Inc.
3803 Bayshore Road
P.O. Box 10096
Palo Alto, CA 94303-0979
1-800-624-1765
650/969-8608 (Fax)
ISBN 0-89016-035-9

APPENDIX

Recommended Responses to Chapter Review Questions

Chapter 1

1. All of the above
2.

Intradisciplinary Teams	Teams are composed of workers from the *same* discipline: registered nurses developing new charting procedures; home health aides coordinating patient visits; insurance claims processors expediting financial reimbursements; and secretaries testing new computer software.
Interdisciplinary Teams	Teams are composed of workers from *different* disciplines: such as registered nurses and dietitians monitoring the progress of diabetic patients; radiographers, laboratory personnel, and admitting clerks streamlining inpatient pre-admission testing; or housekeeping, maintenance, and risk management workers addressing cleanliness and safety issues.
Intradepartmental	Teams are composed of workers from the *same* department: phlebotomists, medical laboratory technicians, and medical technologists reducing the cost of laboratory supplies; pharmacists selecting new drugs; or medical assistants arranging continuing education sessions.
Interdepartmental	Teams are composed of workers from two or more *different* departments: emergency room personnel, cardiac catheterization technologists, and surgical nurses devising methods of getting heart attack victims assessed and into surgery more quickly; and therapists, therapy assistants, and rehabilitation technicians from occupational therapy and radiation therapy coordinating the care and rehabilitation of cancer patients.
Homogeneous	Teams are composed of workers with similar characteristics (training, job titles, scopes of responsibility, and levels of expertise); for examples, see "intradisciplinary" above.
Heterogeneous	Teams are composed of workers with different characteristics; for examples, see "interdisciplinary" above.

3. Work teams meet on a regular, on-going basis as an integral part of the team members' jobs: registered nurses, licensed practical nurses, and nurse assistants exchanging patient information and coordinating work assignments; operating room schedulers and transportation department personnel making sure patients arrive on time for surgery; and admitting department and financial analysts comparing inpatient census rates with monthly projections.

Project teams are short-term, and are assembled to accomplish specific goals within an established period of time: workers from nursing, central supply, and materials management working over the course of one month to compare use of disposable versus nondisposable patient supplies; environmental services workers meeting over the course of two months to test new disinfectants; and medical assistants, infection control personnel, and public health workers meeting for six months to identify options for improving air quality in a community neighborhood health clinic.

Chapter 2

1. Specialist — Workers who provide one function, or a set of similar functions, in one discipline, such as nurses, respiratory care personnel, physical therapists, cardiovascular diagnostic technologists, radiographers, food service workers, patient transporters, housekeepers, central supply technicians, maintenance workers, patient admitting clerks, financial billing personnel, insurance processors, medical records technicians, and secretaries.

   Hospital Restructuring — Reorganizing the structure and function of departments and worker roles to change the model by which patient care is provided.

   Work Redesign — Reorganizing tasks and worker roles to change job responsibilities, and to support hospital restructuring, such as cross-training specialists so they can provide more than one function; and creating roles for extenders to work under the supervision of more highly educated, experienced, and often licensed personnel.

   Cross-training — Acquisition of new or additional skills in the same discipline or in a different discipline from a worker's original skills: nurses cross-trained to draw blood, perform EKG testing, and give routine respiratory treatments; radiographers in a hospital radiology department cross-trained to work in a satellite x-ray facility on a patient care unit or to perform laboratory testing or help with patient assessments; unit secretaries cross-trained to do patient admitting, medical coding, and financial billing; and housekeepers cross-trained to perform basic maintenance duties, ordering and stocking inventory supplies, and transporting patients.

   Multiskilled Workers — Personnel who have been cross-trained to provide more than one function, often in more than one discipline; for examples, see "cross-training" above.

2. Up until the mid 1980s, most hospitals were divided into different departments, each providing a distinct set of patient tests, treatments, or support services. Departments were separate from one another and from nursing units, where inpatients were housed, and hospital staff functioned primarily as specialists.
3. Within the last ten years, many hospitals have decided to restructure and experiment with new ways of delivering patient care as a means of reducing costs, increasing efficiency, and improving patient outcomes.

4. Multiskilled workers provide more than one function, work in more than one area or department, and are more versatile, flexible, and cost-effective than specialists.
5. Examples of multiskilled clinical workers include nurses cross-trained to draw blood, perform EKG testing, and give routine respiratory treatments; department-based radiographers cross-trained to work in a satellite x-ray facility on a patient care unit or to perform laboratory testing or help with patient assessments; medical assistants cross-trained to perform ultrasound procedures and help with outpatient surgery; and clinical workers in outpatient facilities cross-trained to also provide clerical functions.

   Examples of multiskilled clerical workers include unit secretaries cross-trained to do patient admitting, medical coding, and financial billing; and clerical workers in outpatient facilities cross-trained to acquire patient care skills.

   Examples of multiskilled support staff include housekeepers cross-trained to perform basic maintenance duties, ordering and stocking inventory supplies, and transporting patients.
6. Extender — A person with limited expertise and scope of responsibilities who assists in the work of other personnel with greater expertise and broader, higher scopes of responsibilities. This includes patient care assistants or patient care technicians (nurse extenders), nurse practitioners and physician assistants (physician extenders), and rehabilitation technicians (physical and occupational therapist extenders).
7. Restructuring, work redesign, and multiskilling impact the roles of health care workers by reorganizing who does what, and how and where they do it. Jobs and scopes of responsibility change. Workers are expected to become cross-trained, acquire additional skills, work in different locations, and sometimes function as extenders.

Chapter 3

1. Traditionally, when health care workers participated as team members, they did so as specialists and as representatives of their respective discipline, with discipline-specific job titles and scopes of responsibility. Teams were loosely organized, and an ample supply of supervisors and managers were on hand to establish and enforce policies, arrange schedules and work assignments, and help teams solve problems and achieve goals. Today, many team members have team-based job titles and broader scopes of responsibility. With less assistance from supervisors and managers, teams are expected to function with increasing independence, make higher level decisions, and solve more of their own problems.
2. A self-directed work team has a high level of autonomy and responsibility. Team members might be responsible for planning, conducting, evaluating, and controlling the work of the group.
3. Common activities of self-directed work teams include develop work, holiday, and vacation schedules; develop budgets and allocate resources; orient new team members; and conduct peer performance appraisals.
4. Multifunctional or transdisciplinary work teams consist of teams of multiskilled workers whose job responsibilities include more than one function, often in two or more different disciplines, such as patient care assistants who provide nursing, phlebotomy and EKG functions, or unit support technicians with duties in housekeeping, maintenance, and patient transportation.

5. Employers benefit from today's new teams by increases in flexibility, versatility, and productivity of the staff, as well as by enhanced cost-effectiveness in the use of limited resources. Workers benefit from increases in self-esteem, job challenge, job satisfaction, and job security. They also benefit from enhancements in marketability and opportunities for advancement, as well as having more input to how things are done, and a broader perspective on patient care. Patients benefit from improvements in communication, coordination, continuity, and quality of care. Decisions are made more quickly and patient-worker relationships are enhanced.
6. paradigm — A pattern or model.
7. Today's teams represent a new paradigm in health care because they support a new approach to where employees work, what functions they perform, which disciplines in which they work, and how they work with one another.

Chapter 4

1. It is likely you will become multiskilled and function in a team-based job. No matter where you work or what job you perform, expect to serve on many different teams during your career.
2. Aspects of becoming a health care team member includes the:
   - likelihood of being cross-trained or retrained for a team-based job
   - having a job title and job description that reflect a team-based job
   - being evaluated for the contributions you make as an individual and as a team member
   - having your work performance evaluated by other members of your team
   - having your pay raises based, at least in part, on how well your team performs overall
   - serving on more than one team at a time
   - serving on both traditional-type teams as well as today's new types of teams
   - sometimes serving as a leader, other times as a follower
   - experiencing some difficulty changing from functioning as an individual to functioning as a team member
   - need for a different kind of mind-set and new skills in negotiation, conflict resolution, and group dynamics
   - expecting some new challenges, such as turf issues, less supervision, matrix management, and peer pressure
   - expecting your role and your team's role to change and constantly evolve over time
3. Patients are increasing viewed as members of the health care team because they are better informed today than ever before. They have more access to information on diseases, injuries, and treatment options; they ask more questions; and they play a greater role in decision-making and in their day-to-day health care.
4. Because of today's reliance on teams and teamwork, an individual worker's performance appraisal and pay increase may be based, at least in part, on not only how well he or she performs, but also on how well his or her team performs overall.
5. New workers might have less difficulty than experienced workers participating in today's health care teams because experienced workers are used to functioning as individuals (and as specialists) and must now make the transition to working as team members (and often as multiskilled workers.)

6. Occupational Turf — A set of functions or job responsibilities felt to be exclusive to workers in one discipline or occupational category. Cross-training is still controversial among some individuals and groups of professionals who feel their exclusive territory is being invaded by others so multiskilled workers must often have to prove themselves and build trust

Matrix Management — A situation in which employees report to two or more managers from different departments or work units. Service associates on a patient care unit might report to the nurse in charge of the unit, as well as a supervisor from environmental services or facilities management, and unit representatives might report to both a nursing unit manager and a supervisor in medical records or patient billing.

Peer Pressure — Demands placed on an individual by other workers of the same rank and status; conflicts that occur within teams when one person does not do his or her share of the work, fails to show up on time, or calls in sick too often.

Chapter 5

1. Functional — Able to achieve desired outcomes.

Dysfunctional — Impaired; unable to achieve desired outcomes. Because you have a team and a job to do does not necessarily mean the experience will be pleasant or successful. Some teams are so dysfunctional it is a wonder they accomplish anything. On the other hand, a functional team, one composed of people who work well together, can accomplish much more than any single individual.

2. Personal attributes and behaviors important in ensuring team success include:

- likes to work with other people
- high level of self-awareness
- honest
- motivated, dependable, reliable
- shows initiative, accepts responsibility
- follows through on commitments
- arrives on time, ready to work
- shows up for work every day except when sick, injured, or called away by an emergency
- always puts patients first
- volunteers to work holidays and extra hours when possible
- willing to help whenever and wherever needed
- makes personal sacrifices on behalf of patients and team members
- practices professional ethics
- applies the Golden Rule
- keeps private information confidential

- views coworkers as customers
- looks for the good in people
- gives others the benefit of the doubt
- does not spread gossip
- shares information and resources
- helps others learn and build confidence
- praises other people for their accomplishments; gives credit to others
- strives to be part of the solution, not part of the problem
- keeps a positive attitude and sense of humor; laughs at oneself
- is committed to doing a good job

3. Teams need a variety of personality types to be effective. For example, abstract thinkers need practical people to implement their new ideas, and introverts need extroverts to make presentations in front of groups. Although having people with the same personality types on a team might result in less friction, misunderstandings, and disagreements, a variety of different personality types are necessary to see a project through from beginning to end. The challenge is knowing how to best use each person's unique characteristics for the benefit of the entire team.
4. It is important to know your job's parameters and legal scope of practice to be certain you are functioning safely and within legal boundaries. Operating outside your legal scope of practice puts yourself, your patients, coworkers, and employer at risk.
5. Accountability means making sure that the job gets done, either by yourself or someone else. Coordinating team efforts is a challenge. Do not assume that someone else will complete the task.. Saying "that's not my job" is unacceptable. Even if doing the job is not your responsibility, making sure the information is communicated to the right person.
6. Life-long learning means keeping your skills up-to-date. Continuing the learning process is important for health care workers because their most vital contributions to the team are their knowledge, skills, and abilities. They must learn from their mistakes, seize new opportunities for growth, continually strive for quality, and make a commitment to becoming better and better at what they do.
7. Job-related stress can result from a high degree of change, pressures of working in a team-based job, and working with the sick and terminally ill. Team members need stress management skills to help them take care of themselves and protect their own health, and also to provide support for team members and patients.
8. Coping with change means tolerating it. Embracing change means adapting to it, leading it, and looking for ways that change can lead to improvements and new opportunities.
9. Proactive people take action in advance, before the need actually occurs. Reactive people respond and take action after the need has occurred. It is best to be proactive because it enables you to think and plan ahead and anticipate needs before they occur.
10. Good organizational and problem-solving skills are crucial elements of success for individuals and team members. A disorganized approach to work is a major barrier in achieving goals and getting work done efficiently. Health care workers must be able to solve problems efficiently and creatively, address old problems in new ways, and learn to "think out of the box."
11. Interpersonal communication is giving and receiving information through interactions with a variety of people. Poor communication is the leading

cause of interpersonal conflict, misunderstandings, disagreements, arguments, and confrontations with others. Strong interpersonal communication skills give you the tools you need to resolve those kinds of conflicts, and to be an effective team member.

12. Good listening skills and an awareness of body language are important in teamwork because communication is a two-way process. Understanding what the other person is saying is just as important as stating your own message effectively. Active listening shows respect for the other person, and can help prevent misunderstandings that often lead to conflict. Not all communication is verbal. You can tell a lot about how someone feels by their facial expressions and gestures, how they sit or stand, and whether or not they make eye contact with you.

13.

Aggressive	Bold and domineering; disrespectful of the opinions and feelings of others, as in "You idiot! Why do not you learn to drive?"
Passive	Stating no opposition, submissive; devaluing one's own opinion or feelings, as in "I'm so sorry. I'm sure this was all my fault. I just can't seem to do anything right."
Passive-aggressive	Appearing submissive but underhandedly aggressive; dishonest and disrespectful, as in stating the situation is your fault but then secretly doing something to "get even."
Assertive	A positive and confident statement of opinion; respectful of all points of view, as in "I believe I had the right of way, but I'll telephone the police department, and when the officer arrives, we'll ask for clarification."

14. Assertive communication is best because it allows you to state your own views without attacking other people. It is the most effective way to resolve interpersonal conflict because you stand up for yourself while still showing respect for the other person.

15.

Group Dynamics	Tensions, interrelationships, and interactions between two or more people in a group setting.
Consensus	An agreement which is acceptable to everyone.

16. The quiet person, who rarely says anything unless pressured to do so, impedes reaching consensus because all group members need to be full participants.

The person who dominates the discussion and interrupts other people when they have something they want to say themselves, impedes consensus because everyone has a right to be heard and no one person should dominate the discussion.

The "devil's advocate," always critiquing other people's suggestions and questioning their input, impedes consensus because each member should be encouraged to participate.

The harmonizer, who tries to keep everyone happy and make sure all opinions are voiced, supports consensus by building relationships and ensuring that everyone is heard.

The clarifier, who restates what others have said to be certain everyone's clear on the message, supports consensus by helping facilitate effective communication and clearing up any misunderstandings.

The diagnoser, who identifies barriers that keep the group from achieving its goals, supports consensus by helping to identify, and potentially remove, barriers to success.

The clown, who jokes around and distracts the group from its work, impedes consensus by wasting time, and preventing the group from staying focused.

The "blocker," who creates barriers, impedes consensus by "shutting down" communication and prohibiting progress in reaching goals.

"Consensus builders," who poll individuals for their opinions, supports consensus by "testing" the group's progress towards reaching agreement.

17. Examples of cultural differences include age, gender, race, ethnic heritage, lifestyle preference, socioeconomic status, occupational classification, and physical condition.
18. Years ago, people were encouraged to tolerate diversity, but today it is important to value diversity, to understand it, become comfortable with it, and to apply its strengths to benefit everyone.
19. Diversity within a team can sometimes create difficult challenges because cultural differences affect people's values, and the way they approach life and work. But Americans live in a multicultural society, and diversity issues are often at the forefront in health care as you encounter people from all walks of life. Cultural differences within a team can bring a variety of perspectives and add the richness of diversity.
20. Responsibilities of team leaders include serving as a facilitator and coach, organizing and coordinating activities, lining up resources, monitoring efforts of coworkers, tracking progress, and reporting results. Team leaders help solve problems, and make sure everyone has input into decisions and access to the latest information. They identify staff development and training needs, arrange continuing education sessions, lead team meetings, and help manage group dynamics. Being a team leader is not the same as being a supervisor. Supervisors have workers who report to them, and the supervisor is held accountable for the work of subordinates. Team leaders do not have "direct reports," and are not held personally accountable for the performance of their teammates.

Responsibilities of followers include commitment to the job, accepting assignments, following directions, communicating and cooperating with others, and completing tasks on time. Being an effective follower is just as important as being an effective leader because the skills and roles of each person is vital to the overall success of high-performance work teams.

INDEX